Yoga Therapy and Lymphatic System

Evidence-based yogic practices

Boost Your Immune System and Promote Detoxification with Specialized Yoga Practices

Graham Julian Oliver

Copyright © 2024 by Graham Julian Oliver

All rights reserved. No part of this publication may be reproduced, distributed, or transmitted in any form or by any means, including photocopying, recording, or other electronic or mechanical methods, without the prior written permission of the author, except in the case of brief quotations embodied in critical reviews and certain other non-commercial uses permitted by copyright law.

For permission requests, contact the author directly.

Published by Graham Julian Oliver

Disclaimer

This book, *Yoga Therapy and the Lymphatic System: Evidence-Based Yogic Practices - Boost Your Immune System and Promote Detoxification with Specialized Yoga Practices*, is intended solely for informational and educational purposes. It is not a substitute for professional medical advice, diagnosis, or treatment. Always seek the guidance of a qualified healthcare provider with any questions you may have regarding a medical condition or before implementing any new exercise, health program, or wellness regimen.

The content presented in this book is based on evidence-based research and yoga practices intended to support lymphatic health and general wellness. However, individual results may vary, and the author makes no guarantees regarding the effectiveness of the practices discussed for any specific person or health condition. Readers should approach the content with caution and at their own discretion.

The author and publisher expressly disclaim any responsibility or liability for any adverse effects, injuries, or losses that may arise from the application of techniques or suggestions discussed herein. Readers are advised to perform these practices under the supervision of a qualified yoga therapist, especially if they have pre-existing health conditions, injuries, or concerns.

Additionally, the author does not endorse or affiliate with any specific individual, product, website, organization, or any other names that might be referenced or mentioned in this book. All mentions are for informational purposes only. Any similarity to specific therapies, products, or methods is purely incidental.

About This Book

"Yoga Therapy and the Lymphatic System: Evidence-Based Yogic Practices" offers an invaluable guide to the interconnection between specialized yoga practices and lymphatic health, presenting readers with practical, science-backed techniques to support immune function, enhance detoxification, and promote overall wellness. This book opens by grounding readers in a foundational understanding of the lymphatic system's role in detoxification and immunity. It clarifies how lymphatic health is integral to overall well-being and how specific yoga practices can uniquely stimulate lymphatic flow and drainage, distinguishing lymphatic yoga's benefits from those of traditional yoga.

Emphasizing evidence-based yoga therapy, this book is designed with accessibility in mind, guiding readers through safe practices that prioritize lymphatic health from a beginner-friendly perspective. Practical advice on creating a supportive environment, choosing tools, and tracking progress empowers readers to start their journey toward healthier lymphatic function and observe the benefits of consistent practice.

The book thoroughly explains the principles of lymphatic yoga, from understanding its core concepts to incorporating specific poses that stimulate lymphatic flow. By highlighting the importance of deep breathing, stretching, and relaxation, it provides guidance on developing routines that align with each reader's unique needs. Readers will find helpful tips for beginners, warm-up exercises, injury prevention techniques, and options for integrating yoga aids to enrich their practice. Additionally, using visualizations to inspire motivation and mindfulness techniques enhances focus, creating a well-rounded approach to wellness.

A wide array of essential yoga poses specifically aimed at lymphatic health are detailed, each contributing to a comprehensive practice that incorporates breathing exercises and relaxing poses. With an emphasis on breathing techniques for detoxification, readers will explore focused, deep breathing, rhythmic breathing, and techniques like Ujjayi and Kapalabhati. These exercises not only support lymphatic health but also enhance mental clarity and reduce stress, amplifying the impact of the physical practice.

Recognizing the importance of mindfulness, the book introduces meditative techniques that bolster lymphatic function and mental clarity. Guided visualization exercises, stress reduction methods, and practices to enhance focus serve as powerful tools for a holistic experience. This book also introduces seated postures that aid lymphatic flow, encouraging a balance of physical relaxation and mental tranquility. It provides step-by-step guidance on shoulder and neck exercises, chest-opening poses, and mindful breathing, which can easily be incorporated into daily life.

For readers seeking a targeted approach, the book covers upper and lower body practices that support lymphatic activation, circulation, and flexibility. Poses that stimulate blood flow, alleviate tension, and encourage proper lymphatic drainage are methodically outlined, as are detoxifying twists and inversions that aid in toxin release and spinal mobility.

Readers will be empowered to create a personalized routine tailored to their lymphatic health goals. Techniques for balancing poses, incorporating breath work and mindfulness, adjusting for energy levels, and using yoga props help build a fulfilling practice that evolves over time. Common questions about lymphatic yoga and its compatibility with various health conditions are also addressed, providing clear answers on achieving the best results for lasting lymphatic and immune support.

Table of Contents

Introduction

Role of the Lymphatic System in Detoxification and Immunity

The lymphatic system is a critical part of the immune system, responsible for removing toxins, waste, and pathogens from the body. Lymph fluid carries these impurities to lymph nodes, where immune cells neutralize them.

Unlike the circulatory system, which has the heart to pump blood, the lymphatic system relies on body movements and muscle contractions to circulate lymph fluid. Yoga can assist in lymph movement, providing a natural detoxification method by activating key muscles and creating pressure variations that help lymph fluid flow.

Practices like inversions (e.g., legs-up-the-wall) and dynamic poses (such as cat-cow) stimulate lymphatic flow. These movements squeeze and release the lymph nodes, helping to push lymph fluid through the body more effectively. Regular lymph-focused yoga sessions can support immunity by continuously helping the body flush out unwanted substances, thereby reducing the burden on other detoxification organs.

Connection between Lymphatic Health and Overall Wellness

Maintaining lymphatic health is essential for overall wellness, as a stagnant lymph system can lead to fluid retention, reduced immunity, and chronic inflammation. When lymphatic circulation is optimized, the body efficiently eliminates toxins, which helps to balance bodily functions and maintain energy levels. In a healthy lymphatic system, the fluid flows freely, supporting all organs, maintaining healthy skin, and even improving mental clarity by reducing physical toxins.

Yoga's deep breathing exercises, gentle twists, and controlled movements act as a natural pump, enhancing lymph circulation and decreasing lymphatic stagnation. Practices like thoracic breathing (deep belly breaths) combined with postures such as twists or gentle spinal movements can enhance the effect, especially when done daily. This consistent focus on lymph health through yoga boosts overall vitality, helping to keep illnesses at bay and promoting long-term physical wellness.

How Yoga Supports Lymphatic Flow and Drainage

Supporting Lymphatic Flow

Yoga supports lymphatic flow by utilizing a variety of physical movements that compress and release pressure around lymph nodes, located primarily in the neck, underarms, and groin. Movements like inversions, where the head is below the heart, help gravity assist lymph drainage, as lymph flows toward these nodes for filtration. Poses like downward dog, forward fold, and bridge help gently increase circulation, aiding lymphatic return to these nodes for cleansing.

To enhance drainage, practices such as deep breathing and stretching work synergistically to facilitate lymph movement. Practitioners can alternate between gentle flow sequences (e.g., sun salutations) and static holds to boost circulation and lymphatic return effectively.

Regular practice of these techniques creates a rhythmic lymphatic "massage," keeping the flow constant and thereby encouraging detoxification.

Differences between Lymphatic Yoga and Traditional Yoga

Lymphatic-focused yoga specifically targets movements and breath patterns that stimulate the lymphatic system, as opposed to traditional yoga, which focuses more broadly on strength, flexibility, and mental calm. This specialized form of yoga emphasizes low-impact movements and poses that compress lymph nodes and major lymph vessels, using gravity and breathing to aid lymph circulation. By specifically targeting areas where lymph nodes are concentrated, lymphatic yoga supports efficient waste removal from the body.

Unlike traditional yoga, which may involve more intense or sustained poses, lymphatic yoga includes gentle, repetitive movements, often focusing on inversions and joint rotations. Practices are commonly slower-paced, encouraging relaxation and supporting the lymphatic system through subtle yet effective movement, helping maintain the system's balance without over-stressing the body.

Benefits of Lymphatic-Focused Yoga Practices

Detoxification and Immune Boosting

Lymphatic yoga enhances the body's detoxification process by optimizing lymph flow and promoting the removal of toxins. Movements that create rhythmic pressure, such as cat-cow stretches and gentle backbends, massage the lymph nodes, helping to flush out impurities effectively. By incorporating daily lymphatic-focused practices, individuals can support natural detoxification and encourage the body's own defense mechanisms to operate efficiently.

With enhanced lymph circulation, the immune system becomes more effective at filtering out harmful substances. Practices such as deep breathing exercises and gentle flow sequences can be particularly beneficial, as they also help reduce stress—a factor that can negatively impact immunity. By supporting the lymphatic system, yoga assists in maintaining a strong immune response and a clean internal environment.

Getting Started with Evidence-Based Yoga Therapy

Importance of Evidence-Based Yoga in Modern Therapy

Evidence-based yoga integrates scientific research with traditional practices, establishing a framework that validates yoga's benefits for physical and mental health. This approach ensures that yoga therapy is grounded in empirical data, helping practitioners and therapists choose methods that are effective for specific health conditions, including issues related to the lymphatic system. By focusing on evidence-based techniques, individuals can experience enhanced outcomes and a more profound understanding of how yoga supports overall wellness.

Incorporating evidence-based practices into therapy also aids in addressing individual needs. For beginners, starting with simple postures and gradually advancing to more complex sequences allows for a personalized experience. Seeking classes or instructors who prioritize research-backed techniques ensures that practitioners are engaging in practices that are safe and effective, ultimately leading to better health results.

Basics of Practicing Yoga Safely for Lymphatic Health

Practicing yoga safely for lymphatic health involves understanding how specific poses affect the lymphatic system. Gentle movements and restorative postures, such as supported twists and gentle inversions, stimulate lymph flow and promote detoxification. Ensure that you listen to your body and avoid any positions that cause discomfort. Focus on breath work, as deep, diaphragmatic breathing can enhance lymphatic circulation, which is crucial for detoxifying the body.

It is essential to incorporate a warm-up routine to prepare the body before diving into deeper stretches. Simple activities like neck rolls, shoulder shrugs, and ankle rotations can prevent injury and help the lymphatic system function optimally. By gradually introducing these practices into your sessions, you create a safe space for your body to adapt and thrive, enhancing lymphatic health.

How to Build a Consistent, Beginner-Friendly Yoga Routine

Creating a consistent, beginner-friendly yoga routine starts with setting a regular schedule that fits your lifestyle. Aim for short sessions of 20 to 30 minutes, three to four times a week, focusing on foundational poses such as cat-cow, downward-facing dog, and child's pose. These poses are accessible and can be modified based on your flexibility and strength levels. Consistency is key; choose a specific time each day to practice, whether in the morning or evening, to develop a habit.

In addition to physical practice, consider incorporating mindfulness and breathing techniques into your routine. Start or end each session with a few minutes of meditation or deep breathing to cultivate a mind-body connection. This holistic approach not only enhances your physical practice but also fosters mental clarity and relaxation, making it easier to stay committed to your yoga journey.

Choosing the Right Environment and Tools for Practice

Creating an optimal environment for yoga practice involves selecting a space that is quiet, comfortable, and free from distractions. Ideally, your practice area should have good ventilation and be well-lit, allowing natural light to enhance your mood. If possible, use calming elements like plants or soft music to create a serene atmosphere. A dedicated space, even a small corner of a room, can significantly enhance your focus and motivation during practice.

Having the right tools can further improve your experience. Essential items include a yoga mat for grip and comfort, blocks for support, and straps to assist in achieving proper alignment. For beginners, these tools can help modify poses and prevent strain. Additionally, consider using bolsters or blankets for restorative poses to promote relaxation and support, making your practice more enjoyable and effective.

Tracking Your Progress and Feeling the Benefits

To track your progress in yoga, consider maintaining a journal where you note your experiences after each session. Record your feelings, any physical changes, and improvements in flexibility or strength. This reflection not only helps you see how far you've come but also identifies areas where you may want to focus more attention in future practices. Additionally, you can take photos periodically to visually document your journey and celebrate your milestones.

Feeling the benefits of yoga may take time, but being mindful of the subtle changes is crucial. You might notice improved energy levels, better sleep, or decreased stress over time. Pay attention to how your body feels before and after practice, as these observations will reinforce the positive impact of your routine. By acknowledging these benefits, you will stay motivated to continue and deepen your yoga practice.

CHAPTER 1:

The Fundamentals of Lymphatic Yoga

Understanding Lymphatic Yoga Principles

Lymphatic yoga is centered around enhancing lymphatic circulation to support detoxification and immune function. This practice involves gentle movements and specific poses that stimulate the lymph nodes and vessels, promoting better fluid flow. By integrating principles of breath and movement, lymphatic yoga encourages the natural detoxification processes of the body.

To practice lymphatic yoga effectively, it's essential to maintain a calm and mindful approach. Begin with a focus on alignment and slow movements, which can help activate the lymphatic system without strain. Understanding the connection between body posture and lymphatic health will aid in creating a holistic practice that nurtures both physical and mental well-being.

Key Lymphatic-Focused Poses and Their Benefits

Certain yoga poses specifically target the lymphatic system, such as legs-up-the-wall (Viparita Karani), downward dog (Adho Mukha Svanasana), and gentle twists. Legs-up-the-wall promotes venous return and aids lymph drainage, while downward dog encourages the flow of lymph through gravitational effects. Gentle twists stimulate lymph nodes located in the abdomen, further enhancing detoxification.

Incorporating these poses into your practice can yield numerous benefits, including reduced swelling, improved immunity, and increased energy levels. To start, choose a few key poses to focus on, holding each for 5 to 10 breaths, and gradually increase your practice duration as you become more comfortable.

Importance of Deep Breathing for Lymph Flow

Deep breathing plays a crucial role in lymphatic health by facilitating the movement of lymph fluid throughout the body. Engaging in diaphragmatic breathing—where the abdomen expands on the inhale—activates the lymphatic vessels and encourages effective drainage. This technique can significantly enhance the body's detoxification process.

To practice deep breathing, find a comfortable seated position or lie down flat on your back. Place one hand on your abdomen and the other on your chest. Inhale deeply through your nose, allowing your abdomen to rise, and exhale slowly through your mouth. Repeat this for several minutes to promote a relaxed state and stimulate lymph flow.

Stretching and Relaxation for Lymphatic Support

Incorporating stretching and relaxation into your lymphatic yoga practice is vital for maintaining lymphatic health. Gentle stretches can release tension in the body and enhance circulation, aiding in the movement of lymph fluid. Key stretches include neck rolls, side bends, and gentle forward folds.

To practice, dedicate a few minutes at the end of your session to deep stretches, focusing on areas where you feel tightness. Allow your body to relax into each stretch for 30 seconds to a minute, breathing deeply to facilitate the release of tension and support lymphatic circulation.

Ideal Time to Practice Lymphatic Yoga

The ideal time to practice lymphatic yoga varies from person to person, but morning and evening sessions are often beneficial. Practicing in the morning can help invigorate the body and stimulate lymphatic flow, setting a positive tone for the day. Evening sessions can aid in relaxation and detoxification before sleep.

To establish a routine, choose a consistent time that fits your lifestyle, aiming for at least 15 to 30 minutes per session. Listen to your body's needs; if you feel sluggish, opt for a more energetic morning practice, while a gentle evening session can help you unwind.

Simple Warm-Up Exercises for Beginners

Warm-up exercises are essential for preparing the body for lymphatic yoga practice. Simple movements like shoulder rolls, gentle neck stretches, and ankle circles can help release tension and promote blood circulation. These warm-ups activate the lymphatic system without overwhelming beginners.

To begin, stand or sit comfortably and take a few deep breaths. Perform shoulder rolls by lifting your shoulders up towards your ears and then rolling them back and down. Repeat this movement several times, then move to neck stretches by tilting your head side to side, holding each side for a few breaths.

Safety Tips to Avoid Injury

Safety is crucial when practicing lymphatic yoga, especially for beginners. To avoid injury, ensure that your practice space is free from obstacles and that you are using a comfortable mat. Always listen to your body and modify poses as needed to suit your individual abilities.

Additionally, start with shorter sessions and gradually increase duration and intensity as you build strength and flexibility. If you experience pain or discomfort, pause and reassess your alignment and form. Consulting a yoga instructor can also provide personalized guidance and modifications.

Developing a Beginner's Routine

Creating a beginner's routine for lymphatic yoga should include a mix of poses, deep breathing, and relaxation techniques. Start with a few key poses such as legs-up-the-wall, gentle twists, and stretches, aiming for a balanced flow. Include 5 to 10 minutes of deep breathing at the beginning and end of your practice.

To structure your routine, consider spending around 20-30 minutes in total. Begin with a gentle warm-up, then transition into your selected poses, and finish with relaxation and mindfulness. Consistency is key; aim to practice regularly to cultivate familiarity and progress in your practice.

How to Combine Poses for a Full Practice

Combining poses for a full lymphatic yoga practice can create a seamless flow that enhances the benefits of each posture. Start with grounding poses like mountain pose (Tadasana) to establish stability, then flow into poses that promote lymphatic drainage, such as downward dog and side bends.

Create a sequence by linking poses with your breath, transitioning smoothly between each one. For example, move from downward dog to a gentle forward fold (Uttanasana), then into a seated twist. Aim to include a variety of poses that target different areas of the body to support overall lymphatic health

Visualizing the Lymphatic System for Motivation

Visualizing the lymphatic system can enhance your yoga practice by providing motivation and intention. Picture the lymphatic vessels as a network that promotes detoxification and fluid movement throughout the body.

This mental imagery can enhance focus and deepen your practice.

Before beginning your session, take a moment to visualize the lymphatic system at work, imagining the fluid flowing freely and the removal of toxins. This practice of visualization can be particularly effective during deep breathing exercises, reinforcing the connection between breath and lymphatic health.

Using Yoga Blocks and Other Aids

Yoga blocks and other props can significantly enhance your lymphatic yoga practice, providing support and stability. Blocks can help modify poses, making them more accessible for beginners. They can be used to elevate the hands in forward folds or to provide additional support in seated poses.

To incorporate blocks, place one under your hands in downward dog or use it for support in seated forward bends. Other aids like straps can also assist in achieving proper alignment and depth in poses. Don't hesitate to explore different props to find what feels best for your body.

Mindfulness Techniques to Complement the Practice

Integrating mindfulness techniques into your lymphatic yoga practice can deepen the experience and enhance benefits. Techniques like body scanning or focusing on the breath can promote relaxation and heightened awareness of bodily sensations, which can support lymphatic health.

Begin your practice with a few moments of mindfulness by closing your eyes and bringing attention to your breath or doing a quick body scan from head to toe. This intentional focus can ground you in the present moment, helping to cultivate a more enriching practice.

Progress Tracking to Observe Improvements

Tracking your progress in lymphatic yoga can be a motivating and insightful practice. Consider maintaining a journal where you document your sessions, noting how you feel before and after each practice. This can help you observe improvements in your body and mindset over time.

Additionally, keep track of the poses you practice and any changes in flexibility, strength, or energy levels. Regularly reviewing your entries can provide a clearer picture of your journey, helping you celebrate achievements and make adjustments to your routine as needed.

CHAPTER 2:

Essential Yoga Poses for Lymphatic Health

Mountain Pose for Grounding and Balance

Mountain Pose, or Tadasana, serves as the foundation for all standing poses, promoting grounding and balance. To practice, stand tall with your feet hip-width apart, weight evenly distributed. Engage your thighs, lift your chest, and reach your arms overhead with palms facing each other. Hold this position for five breaths, focusing on your breath and allowing your body to feel stable and centered.

This pose encourages awareness of your body's alignment and helps connect you to the earth, fostering a sense of stability. To deepen the practice, close your eyes and visualize your energy flowing down through your feet into the ground. This can enhance your grounding and balance further, making it an excellent starting point for your yoga session.

Downward Dog for Full-Body Activation

Downward Dog, or Adho Mukha Svanasana, is a powerful pose that activates the entire body. Start on your hands and knees, tuck your toes under, and lift your hips toward the ceiling. Your body should form an inverted "V" shape, with your hands shoulder-width apart and feet hip-width apart. Hold this position for five breaths, pressing your heels toward the ground and relaxing your neck.

This pose stretches the spine, hamstrings, and calves while strengthening the arms and shoulders. To enhance the benefits, pedal your feet one at a time to deepen the stretch in your legs. This full-body activation helps stimulate lymphatic circulation, promoting overall detoxification.

Cat-Cow Stretch for Spinal Health

The Cat-Cow stretch is a gentle sequence that promotes spinal flexibility and health. Start on all fours with your wrists aligned under your shoulders and knees under your hips. Inhale, arch your back, and lift your head

(Cow Pose); then exhale, round your spine, and tuck your chin (Cat Pose). Repeat this flow for 5-10 cycles, coordinating your breath with your movements.

This dynamic movement encourages spinal mobility and helps stimulate lymphatic flow through the torso. To enhance the practice, focus on deep, mindful breaths, allowing each movement to release tension and promote relaxation within the spine.

Shoulder Stand to Stimulate Lymph Flow

Shoulder Stand, or Sarvangasana, is an inversion that encourages lymphatic drainage. Lie on your back, lift your legs overhead, and support your lower back with your hands. Your body should form a straight line from shoulders to feet. Hold this pose for 5-10 breaths, allowing gravity to assist in moving lymph toward the heart.

This pose helps stimulate the thyroid and promotes overall hormonal balance while enhancing lymphatic flow. For beginners, it's essential to keep the neck relaxed and avoid straining; using a folded blanket under your shoulders can provide support and comfort.

Spinal Twists to Activate Lymph Nodes

Spinal twists are excellent for activating lymph nodes and promoting detoxification. Sit in a comfortable position with your legs extended. Inhale to lengthen your spine, then exhale and twist your torso to one side, placing your opposite hand on your knee. Hold for 5 breaths and switch sides.

This gentle rotation helps stimulate the digestive system and encourages lymphatic circulation throughout the body. Focus on the breath, using each inhale to lengthen and each exhale to deepen the twist. Incorporating spinal twists into your practice can effectively release tension and support lymphatic health.

Bridge Pose for Chest and Neck Lymph Flow

Bridge Pose, or Setu Bandhasana, opens the chest and stimulates lymph flow in the neck. Lie on your back with your knees bent and feet hip-width apart. Press your feet into the ground and lift your hips toward the ceiling. Interlace your fingers under your back for support and hold for 5-10 breaths.

This pose enhances blood flow to the heart and promotes relaxation in the neck and shoulders. To deepen the benefits, visualize your breath flowing into your heart space as you lift, creating a sense of openness and connection with your body's lymphatic system.

Leg Raises to Promote Leg Lymph Movement

Leg Raises are a simple yet effective way to promote lymphatic movement in the legs. Lie on your back with your legs extended. Inhale deeply and lift your legs to a 90-degree angle, keeping them straight. Hold for a few breaths, then lower them slowly back down without touching the floor.

This exercise encourages circulation and stimulates the lymphatic vessels in the legs, helping to reduce swelling and improve detoxification. To enhance the practice, you can also point and flex your feet while your legs are raised, adding gentle movement to further activate lymph flow.

Inversions for Enhanced Drainage

Inversions, such as Handstand or Headstand, significantly aid lymphatic drainage. Begin in a safe environment and use a wall for support if needed. For a Headstand, start on your knees, interlace your fingers behind your head, and place the crown of your head on the ground. Lift your legs towards the ceiling, holding for 5-10 breaths.

These poses reverse gravity's effects, encouraging lymphatic fluid to flow more freely toward the heart. For beginners, it's crucial to focus on a strong core and controlled movements to prevent injury. Use a wall for support to build confidence as you practice.

Breathing Exercises for Lymph Support

Breathing exercises, or pranayama, are essential for lymphatic support. Start with a simple practice like diaphragmatic breathing. Sit comfortably, place one hand on your abdomen, and inhale deeply through your nose, allowing your belly to expand. Exhale slowly through your mouth, feeling your belly contract. Repeat for several minutes.

This practice helps stimulate lymphatic circulation by encouraging deep, full breaths that promote relaxation and reduce stress. Incorporating breathing techniques into your yoga routine can enhance your overall practice, making it easier for your body to detoxify naturally.

Gentle Backbends for Upper Body Activation

Gentle backbends, like Cobra Pose or Sphinx Pose, activate the upper body and open the chest. To practice Cobra, lie on your stomach with your hands under your shoulders. Inhale, pressing into your palms to lift your chest while keeping your elbows bent. Hold for 5 breaths, feeling the stretch in your chest and shoulders.

These poses encourage the flow of lymphatic fluid in the upper body and can alleviate tension in the back and shoulders. Focus on lengthening the spine and opening the heart center, visualizing breath moving freely through your body.

Svanasana to Integrate the Practice

Svanasana, or Corpse Pose, is vital for integrating your yoga practice. Lie on your back with your arms at your sides and legs comfortably apart. Close your eyes and take deep, calming breaths, allowing your body to relax fully for 5-15 minutes.

This pose helps promote deep relaxation and encourages the body to absorb the benefits of your practice. Use this time to visualize any areas in your body needing lymphatic support, focusing on your breath and allowing your body to rejuvenate and restore.

Child's Pose for Deep Relaxation

Child's Pose, or Balasana, is an excellent restorative pose that promotes deep relaxation. Kneel on the floor, sit back on your heels, and extend your arms forward on the ground. Allow your forehead to rest on the mat and breathe deeply, holding for several breaths.

This pose gently stretches the back, promoting relaxation and lymphatic flow throughout the body. It's a great way to transition between more intense poses and serves as a moment to reconnect with your breath and inner calm.

Visualization to Focus on Lymph Flow

Visualization can enhance your practice by focusing your mind on lymphatic health. While in a comfortable seated position, close your eyes and visualize white light or a flowing stream representing lymphatic fluid circulating through your body. Spend a few moments imagining this fluid flushing out toxins and promoting healing.

Incorporating this technique into your practice can deepen your awareness of lymphatic flow and enhance your overall yoga experience. By focusing on positive imagery, you can create a powerful connection between your mind and body, supporting lymphatic health.

CHAPTER 3:

Breathing Techniques for Enhanced Detoxification

Introduction to Diaphragmatic Breathing

Diaphragmatic breathing, also known as abdominal or belly breathing, involves engaging the diaphragm fully while inhaling. This technique encourages deeper breaths and allows the lungs to fill more completely with air, promoting better oxygen exchange. To practice, sit or lie down in a comfortable position. Place one hand on your chest and the other on your belly. Inhale deeply through your nose, ensuring that your belly rises while your chest remains relatively still. Exhale slowly through your mouth, feeling your belly fall.

This method not only enhances lung function but also helps to reduce stress and anxiety. For beginners, practicing diaphragmatic breathing for just 5–10 minutes daily can improve relaxation and promote a sense of calm. Over time, you can gradually increase the duration as you become more comfortable with the technique.

Benefits of Focused, Deep Breathing for Lymph Health

Deep breathing stimulates lymphatic flow, which is crucial for detoxification and immune function. By engaging the diaphragm, deep breaths create a gentle massage effect on the lymph nodes, aiding in the removal of toxins and waste products from the body. To implement this, focus on breathing deeply and slowly, allowing your body to relax with each exhale.

Incorporating focused, deep breathing into your daily routine can also enhance your overall well-being. Aim to practice this technique during moments of stress or before bed to calm your mind and support lymphatic health. Regular deep breathing can lead to improved energy levels and a stronger immune response.

Practice of Ujjayi Breathing

Ujjayi breathing, often referred to as "victorious breath," involves slightly constricting the throat while inhaling and exhaling, creating a soft ocean-like sound. To practice, sit comfortably and take a deep breath in through your nose, constricting the back of your throat slightly. As you exhale, maintain the constriction, allowing the breath to flow out slowly and audibly. This practice can be combined with yoga postures to enhance focus and concentration.

Ujjayi breathing can calm the nervous system, making it beneficial during yoga or meditation. Aim to incorporate Ujjayi breath into your sessions for 10–15 minutes, focusing on the sound and sensation of your breath. This technique not only helps maintain a steady rhythm but also increases oxygen intake, promoting better lymphatic health.

Rhythmic Breathing for Relaxation

Rhythmic breathing involves establishing a consistent pattern of inhalation and exhalation, which can help induce a state of relaxation. A simple practice is to inhale for a count of four, hold for a count of four, and exhale for a count of four. Start this practice in a quiet space, allowing your breath to naturally guide your body into a relaxed state.

As you become more comfortable, experiment with extending the counts, such as inhaling for six and exhaling for six, to deepen your relaxation. Rhythmic breathing can be particularly effective when feeling stressed or anxious, providing a grounding effect that calms the mind and body.

Alternate Nostril Breathing for Balance

Alternate nostril breathing, or Nadi Shodhana, is a pranayama technique that helps balance the body and mind by harmonizing the right and left hemispheres of the brain. Begin by sitting comfortably and closing your right nostril with your right thumb. Inhale deeply through your left nostril, then close it with your ring finger. Open your right nostril and exhale through it. Inhale through the right nostril, close it, and exhale through the left. Repeat this pattern for several minutes.

This practice can enhance mental clarity and reduce stress. It's ideal to practice alternate nostril breathing for 5–10 minutes daily, especially during times of emotional turmoil or when you seek balance. The calming effect it provides can significantly improve your overall well-being.

Kapalabhati for Energizing and Detox

Kapalabhati, or "skull shining breath," is a powerful pranayama technique designed to energize the body and cleanse the lungs. To practice, sit comfortably with a straight spine. Inhale deeply, then exhale forcefully through your nose while pulling your belly in toward your spine. Allow the inhalation to happen naturally between each forceful exhale. Start with 20-30 rounds and gradually increase as you become more comfortable.

Kapalabhati not only stimulates the digestive system but also increases oxygen flow to the brain, enhancing mental clarity. Incorporating this practice into your morning routine can help detoxify the body and boost energy levels, making it a refreshing way to start your day.

Timing and Duration of Breathing Exercises

When starting your breathing exercises, consider dedicating 5–15 minutes daily. It's important to find a time that suits you best—whether in the morning to start your day or in the evening to wind down. Begin with simple exercises like diaphragmatic breathing or rhythmic breathing, and gradually increase the duration and complexity as you become more comfortable.

Establishing a routine helps build consistency and reinforces the benefits of your practice. Listen to your body and adjust the timing according to your personal needs. As you progress, you can experiment with different durations, allowing you to find the balance that works best for you.

Combining Breathwork with Yoga Poses

Integrating breathwork with yoga poses enhances the overall benefits of both practices. As you flow through yoga postures, coordinate your breath with movement—for instance, inhaling while raising your arms and exhaling while folding forward. This synchronicity not only helps deepen your stretches but also promotes relaxation and mindfulness during practice.

To start, choose a few simple poses, such as Cat-Cow or Downward Dog, and incorporate specific breathing techniques, like Ujjayi or diaphragmatic breathing. By connecting breath and movement, you can enhance the effectiveness of your practice and support your lymphatic health.

Safety Tips for Beginners in Pranayama

For beginners, it's essential to approach pranayama with mindfulness and care. Always practice in a comfortable position and avoid forcing your breath; let it flow naturally. Start with simple techniques, gradually increasing complexity as you gain confidence. Ensure you're in a well-ventilated space to enhance oxygen intake.

If you experience any discomfort, dizziness, or shortness of breath, immediately stop the practice and return to normal breathing. Consulting with a yoga instructor or healthcare professional can provide guidance tailored to your individual needs, ensuring a safe and beneficial experience.

Effects of Oxygen Flow on Lymph Nodes

Deep, controlled breathing enhances oxygen flow throughout the body, positively impacting the lymphatic system. Increased oxygen levels can stimulate lymph node function, promoting detoxification and immune health. As you breathe deeply, your body becomes more effective at filtering out waste and toxins, leading to better overall wellness.

To maximize these benefits, practice deep breathing techniques regularly, focusing on the quality of each inhalation and exhalation. Simple exercises, such as diaphragmatic breathing, can create a significant positive impact on lymphatic health over time.

Breathing to Release Toxins and Boost Immunity

Focused breathing techniques can aid in releasing toxins and boosting immunity. By enhancing oxygen supply, you enable your body to detoxify more efficiently. For instance, Kapalabhati and Ujjayi breathing stimulate the respiratory and lymphatic systems, encouraging the expulsion of waste products.

Incorporating these practices into your daily routine helps to strengthen your immune system. Aim to engage in specific breathing exercises, especially after illness or during high-stress periods, to support your body's natural detoxification processes.

Relaxation Between Breath Exercises

Allowing time for relaxation between breath exercises is crucial for maximizing benefits. After completing a series of breathwork techniques, take a moment to return to normal breathing and observe how your body feels. This can enhance the effects of the exercises and provide a greater sense of calm and clarity.

You can also incorporate gentle stretches or a brief meditation during these relaxation periods to further deepen your experience. This approach fosters a more holistic practice, helping you to integrate the benefits of breathwork into your overall well-being.

Monitoring Your Progress

Tracking your progress in breathwork and yoga can help you stay motivated and identify improvements in your practice. Consider maintaining a journal to record your experiences, noting any changes in how you feel physically and emotionally. This can include details such as your breathing techniques, duration of practice, and overall energy levels.

As you continue, reflect on your journey and celebrate milestones, no matter how small. Monitoring progress not only reinforces the habit but also allows you to appreciate the positive effects of your practice on your lymphatic health and overall well-being.

CHAPTER 4:

Seated Postures for Lymphatic Flow

Easy Pose for Meditative Focus

To practice Easy Pose, find a comfortable seated position on the floor with your legs crossed. Sit up tall, ensuring your spine is straight and shoulders are relaxed. Rest your hands on your knees, palms facing up or down. Focus on your breath, inhaling deeply through your nose and exhaling gently through your mouth. This position encourages a calm and centered mindset, making it easier to enter a meditative state.

While in Easy Pose, try to maintain a soft gaze or close your eyes. If your mind begins to wander, gently bring your attention back to your breath or a mantra. Practicing this pose for 5-10 minutes daily can significantly enhance your ability to concentrate and maintain a peaceful mind.

Lotus Pose for Mental Calmness

To get into Lotus Pose, begin seated in Easy Pose, then carefully place each foot on the opposite thigh. Ensure that your knees are resting on the ground, and your spine remains upright. You may use a cushion or blanket underneath you for added support. This pose can create a feeling of stability and grounding, fostering mental calmness and serenity.

While in Lotus Pose, focus on your breathing and try to visualize a peaceful environment. Hold this position for a few minutes, deepening your breath with each exhale. If you find it uncomfortable, consider modifying the pose by keeping one foot on the opposite calf or using the Easy Pose instead.

Cobbler's Pose for Inner Leg Activation

To perform Cobbler's Pose, sit on the floor with the soles of your feet together, allowing your knees to fall outward. Hold your feet with your hands, and sit up tall, elongating your spine. This pose activates the inner thigh muscles and opens the hips, enhancing flexibility and circulation.

While in this pose, gently press your knees towards the floor for a deeper stretch, but don't force them down. Breathe deeply for 5-10 breaths, focusing on releasing any tension in the hips. You can also gently rock your body forward and backward to further engage the inner legs.

Seated Forward Fold for Spinal Stretch

To perform Seated Forward Fold, sit with your legs extended straight in front of you. Inhale and lengthen your spine, then exhale as you hinge at the hips to reach for your feet or shins. Keep your back straight and avoid rounding your shoulders. This pose stretches the spine and hamstrings, promoting relaxation.

While holding the pose, focus on your breath, allowing each exhale to deepen the stretch. Hold for 5-10 breaths, feeling the tension release from your back and legs. If your hands do not reach your feet, use a strap around your feet or place your hands on your shins.

Staff Pose for Grounding

To practice Staff Pose, sit on the floor with your legs extended straight in front of you, feet flexed. Keep your spine straight and place your hands flat on the floor beside your hips. This pose helps create a grounded feeling and promotes stability while strengthening the core and back muscles.

While in this pose, focus on your breath and visualize yourself rooted to the ground. Hold for 5-10 breaths, ensuring your shoulders are relaxed and your chest is open. To increase engagement, try gently pressing your hands into the ground for added stability.

Head-to-Knee Forward Bend for Leg Flexibility

To get into Head-to-Knee Forward Bend, sit with one leg extended and the other foot against your inner thigh. Inhale to lengthen your spine, then exhale as you fold forward over the extended leg. Reach for your foot or shin while keeping your back straight. This pose enhances leg flexibility and stretches the spine.

As you hold the pose, focus on deepening your breath and relaxing into the stretch. Hold for 5-10 breaths, then switch legs. This practice helps improve overall flexibility and encourages relaxation in the body.

Butterfly Stretch for Lower Body Lymph Nodes

To perform Butterfly Stretch, sit with the soles of your feet together and your knees dropped out to the sides. Hold your feet with your hands and sit up tall. This pose opens the hips and stimulates the lymphatic system, which is essential for detoxification.

While in this pose, gently press your knees toward the ground for a deeper stretch. Breathe deeply for 5-10 breaths, feeling the stretch in your inner thighs and hips. This can help improve circulation and promote the flow of lymphatic fluid.

Twist Pose to Release Tension

For Twist Pose, sit with your legs extended in front of you. Bend your right knee and place your foot on the outside of your left thigh. Inhale and lengthen your spine, then exhale as you twist your torso to the right.

Use your left elbow against your right knee to deepen the twist. This pose helps release tension in the spine and promotes digestion.

As you hold the twist, focus on your breath, feeling each inhale lengthen your spine and each exhale deepen the twist. Hold for 5-10 breaths before switching sides. This practice can help relieve back pain and improve spinal mobility.

Reclined Twist for Deep Relaxation

To practice Reclined Twist, lie on your back with your knees bent. Allow your knees to drop to one side while keeping your shoulders flat on the ground. Extend your arms out to the sides in a T-shape. This pose encourages relaxation and aids in detoxifying the body by stimulating the digestive organs.

While in the twist, breathe deeply, focusing on releasing tension in your lower back. Hold for 5-10 breaths, then gently bring your knees back to center and switch sides. This gentle twist helps improve spinal flexibility and promotes overall relaxation.

Spinal Stretch for Lymphatic Movement

For Spinal Stretch, sit cross-legged or in a comfortable seated position. Inhale to lengthen your spine, then exhale as you gently lean to one side, reaching your arm overhead. This pose stretches the spine and opens the side body, encouraging lymphatic flow.

As you hold the stretch, focus on your breath, allowing each inhale to create space in your spine. Hold for 5-10 breaths before switching sides. This practice helps maintain spinal health and promotes overall well-being.

Sitting in Stillness for Meditation

To practice sitting in stillness, find a comfortable seated position, either on the floor or in a chair. Close your eyes and bring your attention to your breath, allowing thoughts to come and go without judgment. This practice encourages mindfulness and mental clarity.

As you sit in stillness, aim to maintain a quiet, focused mind for 5-10 minutes. When distractions arise, gently guide your attention back to your breath. This simple practice can help reduce stress and promote a sense of inner peace.

Guided Breathing with Seated Poses

To incorporate guided breathing, sit comfortably in any seated position. Inhale deeply through your nose, allowing your abdomen to expand, then exhale through your mouth, emptying your lungs. Repeat this for several minutes, synchronizing your breath with gentle movements, such as raising your arms overhead on the inhale and lowering them on the exhale.

While practicing guided breathing, focus on the sensations in your body and the rhythm of your breath. This technique enhances mindfulness and can help reduce anxiety, making it a valuable tool in your yoga practice.

Relaxation Tips for Seated Practices

For effective relaxation during seated practices, ensure your seating is comfortable, using props like cushions or blankets to support your body. Close your eyes, take a few deep breaths, and consciously relax each part of your body, starting from your head and moving down to your toes.

Incorporate gentle movements, such as shoulder rolls or neck stretches, to release tension. Set an intention for your practice, and allow yourself to be fully present, dedicating 5-10 minutes to unwind and rejuvenate your body and mind.

CHAPTER 5:

Incorporating Mindfulness and Meditation

Importance of Mindfulness in Yoga Therapy

Mindfulness in yoga therapy fosters a deep connection between the mind and body, enabling practitioners to be present and aware of their thoughts, feelings, and sensations. This awareness helps in identifying stressors and emotional blockages that can impede the lymphatic system's functioning. By cultivating mindfulness, individuals can respond to their body's needs more effectively, enhancing overall wellness and promoting a healthier lymphatic flow.

To practice mindfulness, begin by dedicating a few minutes daily to focus on your breath. Sit comfortably, close your eyes, and bring your attention to your inhales and exhales. Whenever your mind wanders, gently guide it back to your breath, allowing yourself to embrace the present moment. This simple practice can significantly improve your mental clarity and emotional resilience, benefiting both your mind and lymphatic health.

Introduction to Lymph-Focused Meditation

Lymph-focused meditation emphasizes activating and supporting the lymphatic system through specific meditative practices. This form of meditation not only enhances relaxation but also aids in detoxification, helping to flush out toxins and improve overall health. By concentrating on lymphatic flow, practitioners can encourage better circulation and boost their immune system.

To get started, find a quiet space where you can sit or lie comfortably. Begin by visualizing the lymphatic system—imagine the lymph fluid flowing through your body, cleansing and rejuvenating every cell. Focus on areas where you feel tension or discomfort, and with each breath, visualize the lymphatic fluid gently releasing toxins and promoting healing. Regular practice can lead to enhanced lymphatic health and increased vitality.

Guided Visualization for Lymphatic Health

Guided visualization is a powerful tool that harnesses the imagination to support lymphatic health. By mentally picturing your lymphatic system at work, you can create a sense of empowerment and promote positive bodily changes. This practice is especially beneficial for those seeking to reduce stress and enhance the immune response.

To practice guided visualization, close your eyes and take a few deep breaths. Imagine a serene environment, like a peaceful forest or a tranquil beach. Visualize your lymphatic system as a network of gentle streams, flowing smoothly and effortlessly. As you breathe deeply, imagine these streams carrying away toxins and nourishing your body with healing energy. Engage in this visualization regularly to foster a sense of well-being and vitality.

Techniques for Stress Reduction

Effective stress reduction techniques are essential for maintaining a healthy lymphatic system, as stress can hinder lymphatic flow and immune function. Incorporating simple practices such as deep breathing, gentle yoga, and progressive muscle relaxation can significantly alleviate stress levels.

To reduce stress, start by practicing deep breathing. Inhale deeply through your nose, allowing your abdomen to expand, and then exhale slowly through your mouth. Repeat this for a few minutes, focusing on the sensation of your breath. Additionally, consider integrating gentle yoga stretches that target the neck, shoulders, and back, releasing tension and promoting relaxation.

Benefits of Mental Clarity on Lymphatic System

Achieving mental clarity is crucial for optimal lymphatic function, as a clear mind allows for better decision-making and self-awareness regarding health choices. Improved mental clarity can reduce anxiety and stress, both of which negatively impact the lymphatic system.

To enhance mental clarity, engage in activities that stimulate your mind, such as puzzles, reading, or learning new skills. Pair these activities with regular yoga practices that emphasize focus and concentration, like balancing poses or mindfulness exercises. This combination can create a harmonious connection between your mental and physical well-being, ultimately benefiting your lymphatic health.

5-Minute Meditation Routine for Beginners

A simple 5-minute meditation routine can be an excellent starting point for beginners looking to enhance their lymphatic health. This short practice can help ground your thoughts, reduce stress, and improve awareness of bodily sensations, fostering a healthier lymphatic system.

Begin by finding a comfortable seated position with your spine straight. Set a timer for five minutes, close your eyes, and take a few deep breaths. Focus on your breath, allowing thoughts to come and go without judgment. If your mind wanders, gently bring your attention back to your breath. By establishing this routine, you'll create a foundation for deeper meditation practices in the future.

Techniques to Improve Focus

Improving focus is essential for maintaining mindfulness and enhancing the effectiveness of yoga therapy. Techniques such as setting specific goals, breaking tasks into manageable steps, and minimizing distractions can help sharpen your concentration and promote a clearer mind.

To enhance your focus, try the Pomodoro Technique: work for 25 minutes on a task, then take a 5-minute break. During your breaks, engage in a brief mindfulness exercise, such as deep breathing or stretching. Additionally, consider practicing yoga poses that require concentration, like tree pose or warrior III, to train your mind and body to stay present.

Setting Intentions for Wellness

Setting intentions for wellness allows you to clarify your health goals and create a positive mindset. Intentions serve as a guide for your yoga practice and overall lifestyle choices, helping you stay focused on achieving your desired outcomes for both physical and mental well-being.

To set an intention, find a quiet space and take a few deep breaths. Reflect on what you want to achieve in your wellness journey—whether it's increased energy, reduced stress, or improved lymphatic health. Write your intention down and revisit it regularly, especially before your yoga practice, to reinforce your commitment to your goals.

Practicing Gratitude as a Mindfulness Tool

Practicing gratitude is a powerful mindfulness tool that can enhance mental well-being and support a healthy lymphatic system. Focusing on what you are grateful for can shift your mindset from stress to positivity, creating a more resilient emotional state.

To incorporate gratitude into your daily routine, keep a gratitude journal. Each day, write down three things you are thankful for, no matter how small. This practice not only fosters a positive outlook but also encourages mindfulness as you reflect on your experiences. Over time, you may notice improvements in your overall mood and a more profound connection to your body.

Observing Bodily Sensations for Awareness

Observing bodily sensations enhances awareness and promotes a deeper connection between the mind and body, crucial for supporting lymphatic health. By tuning into how your body feels, you can identify areas of tension and areas needing care, fostering a more responsive approach to your well-being.

To practice this awareness, take a few moments during your yoga session or throughout the day to check in with your body. Close your eyes and focus on different parts, noticing any sensations or areas of discomfort. Acknowledge these feelings without judgment, allowing yourself to explore their origin. This practice will help you develop a more profound awareness of your body's needs and responses.

How to Meditate Anywhere, Anytime

Meditation doesn't have to be confined to a specific space or time; you can practice it anywhere, anytime. This flexibility allows you to incorporate mindfulness into your daily routine, enhancing your lymphatic health and overall wellness regardless of your environment.

To meditate on the go, simply find a comfortable position, whether seated or standing, and focus on your breath. Allow yourself to take a few deep inhales and exhales, tuning into the rhythm of your breath. If you feel overwhelmed or anxious, practice a mini-meditation by counting your breaths—inhale for four counts, hold for four, and exhale for four. This practice can be done in just a few moments during your day, helping to center you wherever you are.

Mindful Breathing as a Quick Reset

Mindful breathing is an effective technique to quickly reset your mental state and support your lymphatic system. By focusing on your breath, you can alleviate stress and create a sense of calm, making it easier to stay present and engaged in your daily activities.

To practice mindful breathing, find a comfortable position and take a deep breath in through your nose, filling your lungs completely. Hold for a moment, then slowly exhale through your mouth. Repeat this cycle several times, paying attention to how your body feels with each breath. Incorporating this simple practice throughout your day can help you maintain a state of mindfulness and improve your overall well-being.

Journaling to Track Progress

Journaling is an invaluable tool for tracking your progress in yoga therapy and enhancing your understanding of your body and mind. This practice encourages reflection on your experiences, helping you identify patterns in your emotions, physical sensations, and lymphatic health over time.

To start journaling, set aside a few minutes each day to write about your thoughts, feelings, and experiences related to your yoga practice. Consider noting any changes you observe in your body or mood, particularly regarding your lymphatic health. Regularly reviewing your entries can provide insights into your growth, helping you stay motivated on your wellness journey.

CHAPTER 6:

Upper Body Practices for Lymphatic Activation

Shoulder Stretches to Relieve Tension

To relieve tension in the shoulders, begin by sitting or standing comfortably with your back straight. Inhale deeply, then raise your shoulders towards your ears, holding the position for a few seconds before exhaling and dropping them down. Repeat this process 5-10 times to encourage relaxation and release tightness. You can also incorporate lateral stretches by bringing one arm overhead while leaning to the opposite side, feeling the stretch along the side of your body.

For a more dynamic stretch, extend your arms out to the sides and gently rotate them in small circles for about 30 seconds. Gradually increase the size of the circles as you feel more comfortable. This helps to increase blood flow and flexibility in the shoulder area, relieving stiffness and enhancing mobility.

Neck Exercises for Lymph Nodes Activation

To activate lymph nodes in the neck, start by sitting up straight and gently tilting your head to one side, bringing your ear towards your shoulder. Hold this position for 15-30 seconds while taking deep breaths, then switch to the other side. This exercise helps stimulate lymphatic circulation and relieve tension in the neck muscles.

Additionally, perform chin tucks by drawing your chin in towards your neck, which strengthens the muscles that support proper posture. Hold the tuck for 5 seconds and repeat 10 times. This exercise not only activates lymph nodes but also helps maintain neck alignment and reduces stiffness.

Arm Movements for Fluid Drainage

Begin fluid drainage exercises by extending your arms overhead and then bending your elbows to bring your hands behind your head. Hold this position for a few breaths, feeling the stretch in your arms and shoulders. Next, slowly lower your arms and perform arm circles to encourage lymphatic flow, moving your arms forward and backward for 30 seconds each.

You can also try the "Windmill" exercise by extending your arms out to the sides and gently twisting your torso to touch your opposite hand to your opposite foot. This motion promotes fluid drainage while engaging your core muscles, enhancing overall mobility.

Chest Openers for Enhanced Breathing

To open up the chest and enhance breathing, stand or sit with your back straight. Interlace your fingers behind your back and straighten your arms while lifting your chest towards the ceiling. Hold for 15-30 seconds, feeling the expansion in your chest. This stretch improves lung capacity and promotes better oxygenation.

Additionally, practice a doorway stretch by placing your arms against a wall or door frame and leaning forward slightly. This movement allows for a gentle opening of the chest, facilitating deeper breaths. Hold this position for 20-30 seconds while focusing on your breath to enhance relaxation.

Shoulder Rolls to Improve Mobility

Shoulder rolls are a simple yet effective exercise for improving mobility. Start by sitting or standing comfortably with your arms relaxed at your sides. Inhale as you roll your shoulders up towards your ears, then exhale as you roll them back and down. Repeat this sequence 10 times in a forward direction, then switch to rolling them backward.

For an added challenge, you can perform shoulder rolls with your arms extended out to the sides. This increases the range of motion and enhances muscle engagement. Incorporate deep breathing to help release any tension stored in the shoulders during the exercise.

Clasped Hands Stretch for Chest Area

To perform the clasped hands stretch, stand or sit with your spine straight. Interlace your fingers and extend your arms straight in front of you, then lift your arms overhead while maintaining the clasp. Hold for 15-30 seconds, feeling the stretch across your chest and shoulders. This position helps to counteract slouching and promotes good posture.

You can also modify this stretch by leaning to one side while keeping your hands clasped overhead. This variation targets the side body and deepens the stretch in the chest area. Breathe deeply and hold the stretch for several breaths before switching sides.

Simple Neck Tilts to Release Stiffness

Begin with simple neck tilts by sitting or standing tall. Slowly tilt your head to one side, bringing your ear towards your shoulder while keeping the opposite shoulder relaxed. Hold this position for 15-30 seconds, then switch sides. This exercise gently stretches the neck muscles and can help alleviate stiffness.

For a deeper stretch, interlace your fingers and place your hands on the back of your head. Apply gentle pressure to encourage a deeper tilt while keeping your shoulders down. Hold for several deep breaths to enhance relaxation and release tension.

Cobra Pose to Open Up the Chest

To practice the Cobra pose, start by lying on your stomach with your legs extended and hands placed under your shoulders. As you inhale, press your hands into the ground, lifting your chest while keeping your elbows slightly bent. Hold the pose for 15-30 seconds, focusing on opening the chest and stretching the abdominal muscles. This position promotes lung expansion and relieves tension in the back.

For a deeper stretch, you can gradually straighten your arms to lift your chest higher. Ensure you keep your shoulders relaxed away from your ears. Remember to breathe deeply, allowing your body to relax into the pose as you enhance your chest opening.

Extended Arm Poses for Circulation

Extended arm poses are excellent for promoting circulation. Begin by standing with your feet hip-width apart and extending your arms overhead, palms facing each other. Hold this position for 15-30 seconds while engaging your core and focusing on your breath. This pose stimulates blood flow and encourages lymphatic drainage.

To deepen the stretch, gently lean to one side, feeling the stretch along the side of your body. Hold for a few breaths, then switch sides. This variation not only enhances circulation but also promotes flexibility and balance in the upper body.

Seated Chest Opener for Flexibility

Start the seated chest opener by sitting cross-legged or on a chair with your feet flat on the ground. Inhale deeply, and as you exhale, interlace your fingers behind your back while lifting your chest. Hold this position for 20-30 seconds to feel the stretch across your chest and shoulders, enhancing flexibility.

To increase the effectiveness of this stretch, you can gently lean forward while keeping your clasped hands lifted. This modification deepens the stretch and further opens up the chest area. Focus on your breath, allowing any tension to release as you maintain the position.

Slow Shoulder Shrugs to Ease Tension

For slow shoulder shrugs, sit or stand comfortably with your arms at your sides. Inhale deeply and lift your shoulders towards your ears. Hold for a moment, then exhale as you drop them down. Repeat this movement 5-10 times to help release accumulated tension in the shoulder area and promote relaxation.

You can also enhance this practice by incorporating deep breathing. As you lift your shoulders, inhale deeply, and as you lower them, exhale slowly. This combination helps to calm the nervous system and encourages a sense of relaxation throughout the body.

Combining with Deep Breathing

Incorporating deep breathing into your yoga practice is essential for enhancing relaxation and detoxification. Begin by sitting comfortably with your hands on your knees or in your lap. Close your eyes and take a deep breath in through your nose, filling your lungs fully. Hold the breath for a moment, then exhale slowly through your mouth. Repeat this cycle for 5-10 breaths, focusing on the rhythm of your breath.

You can also practice deep breathing while performing stretches or poses. For instance, inhale as you reach into a pose and exhale as you release tension. This practice enhances the mind-body connection and promotes a calming effect throughout your yoga routine.

Gentle Twists for Upper Body Relief

To perform gentle twists, sit or stand with a straight spine. Inhale deeply, and as you exhale, twist your torso to one side, placing your hand on your knee or the back of your chair for support. Hold this position for several breaths, feeling the gentle stretch in your spine and upper body. This movement encourages spinal mobility and aids in lymphatic drainage.

After holding the twist for a few breaths, return to the center and switch to the opposite side. Ensure your movements are slow and controlled, allowing your body to ease into the twist. This practice not only helps relieve tension but also stimulates digestion and promotes overall well-being.

CHAPTER 7:

Lower Body Poses for Improved Circulation

Knee-to-Chest Poses for Blood Flow

Knee-to-chest poses are essential for enhancing blood circulation and stimulating the lymphatic system. To perform this pose, lie on your back and bring your knees toward your chest, wrapping your arms around your shins. Hold this position for several breaths, feeling the stretch in your lower back and hips. This pose not only promotes blood flow but also helps to reduce tension in the lower body.

To deepen the stretch, gently rock side to side while maintaining the position, which can enhance relaxation and circulation. This movement can help clear any blockages in the lymphatic pathways, promoting overall detoxification. Aim to hold the pose for 30 seconds to a minute, allowing your body to fully engage in the benefits.

Leg Stretches to Enhance Lymphatic Flow

Leg stretches are vital for stimulating lymphatic flow and improving overall circulation. Simple stretches like hamstring stretches or quad stretches can be done while standing or seated. For a hamstring stretch, sit with one leg extended and reach towards your toes, holding the stretch for 20-30 seconds before switching sides. This helps to open up the hips and promote fluid movement in the legs.

For quadriceps, stand on one leg, pulling the opposite foot towards your glutes, ensuring your knees are aligned. This stretch not only enhances lymphatic drainage but also prepares the body for more dynamic movements. Incorporate these stretches into your daily routine to promote better blood circulation and lymphatic health.

Reclined Bound Angle Pose for Groin Lymph Nodes

Reclined Bound Angle Pose is an effective way to target the lymph nodes in the groin area. To perform this pose, lie on your back and bring the soles of your feet together, allowing your knees to fall out to the sides. This position opens the hips and creates space for lymphatic flow around the groin. Hold this pose for 1-3 minutes, breathing deeply to enhance relaxation.

To increase the effectiveness of this pose, you can place cushions or blocks under your knees for added support. This will allow you to relax deeper into the stretch, facilitating better lymphatic circulation. Practicing this pose regularly can help maintain healthy lymph nodes and promote detoxification.

Forward Fold for Overall Relaxation

The Forward Fold pose is excellent for releasing tension and promoting relaxation throughout the body. To execute this pose, stand tall and hinge at your hips to fold forward, allowing your upper body to hang heavy. You can bend your knees slightly if needed, ensuring you don't strain your lower back. Hold this position for 30 seconds, breathing deeply to release any stress.

To enhance the benefits, you can sway gently side to side or grab opposite elbows for a deeper stretch. This movement encourages lymphatic flow through the legs and lower back, aiding in detoxification. Make this pose a part of your daily routine to help calm the mind and relieve tension.

Standing Splits to Stimulate Legs

The Standing Splits pose stimulates the legs and encourages lymphatic drainage. To perform this pose, begin in a forward fold and then shift your weight onto one leg while raising the other leg straight behind you. Keep your torso hinged forward and your hips squared. Hold for several breaths, focusing on lengthening your lifted leg while grounding through your standing leg.

To deepen the pose, you can place your hands on the floor or use blocks for added support. This will help activate the leg muscles and encourage circulation in the lower body. Practicing Standing Splits can enhance flexibility and promote a healthy lymphatic system.

Gentle Lunges for Leg Activation

Gentle lunges are a simple yet effective way to activate the legs and stimulate lymphatic flow. Start in a standing position, step forward with one foot, and lower your hips into a lunge, ensuring your front knee is aligned with your ankle. Hold this position for a few breaths before switching legs. This movement opens up the hips and encourages fluid movement in the lymphatic system.

For added benefits, you can incorporate upper body movements, like raising your arms overhead as you lunge. This full-body engagement not only promotes lymphatic drainage but also enhances balance and stability. Aim for 5-10 lunges on each side to fully activate your legs and boost circulation.

Tree Pose to Build Balance

Tree Pose is a fantastic balance exercise that strengthens the legs and promotes lymphatic flow. To perform this pose, stand on one leg and place the sole of the opposite foot against your inner thigh or calf, avoiding the knee. Once stable, bring your hands together at your heart or reach them overhead. Focus on a single point in front of you to help maintain your balance.

Holding Tree Pose for 30 seconds to a minute allows your body to engage core muscles while enhancing circulation. As you breathe deeply, visualize energy flowing through your body, promoting lymphatic health. Incorporate this pose into your routine to improve balance and boost overall well-being.

Extended Triangle Pose for Alignment

Extended Triangle Pose is beneficial for improving alignment and stimulating lymphatic flow. To begin, stand with your feet wide apart, turning one foot out. Reach your arm towards the extended foot while the other arm reaches upward, creating a straight line from one hand to the other. Keep your body aligned and engage your core. Hold this position for several breaths.

To deepen the pose, you can look up at your top hand, which will open your chest further. This pose not only stretches the legs and hips but also promotes drainage from the lymph nodes in the groin. Practice Extended Triangle Pose regularly to enhance your overall posture and support lymphatic health.

Pigeon Pose for Hip Flexibility

Pigeon Pose is excellent for increasing hip flexibility and promoting lymphatic drainage. Begin in a tabletop position, bringing one knee forward while extending the opposite leg straight back. Lower your torso down towards the floor, either resting on your forearms or fully extending. Hold this position for 30 seconds to a minute, breathing deeply to release tension.

To enhance the stretch, you can place a cushion under your hip for added support. This pose opens the hips and stimulates the lymphatic system, promoting overall detoxification. Regularly practicing Pigeon Pose can help maintain flexibility and encourage healthy lymphatic flow.

Reclining Big Toe Pose for Leg Stretch

Reclining Big Toe Pose is an effective way to stretch the legs while promoting lymphatic drainage. To perform this pose, lie on your back and extend one leg towards the ceiling, grabbing your big toe or using a strap to assist. Keep the other leg extended on the ground. Hold this position for 30 seconds, feeling the stretch in your hamstrings and calves.

To deepen the stretch, you can gently pull your leg towards your chest, ensuring your back remains flat on the floor. This pose not only enhances flexibility but also promotes blood flow to the legs and supports the lymphatic system. Incorporate this pose into your routine for improved leg strength and lymphatic health.

Calf Raises for Improved Circulation

Calf raises are a simple yet effective exercise for boosting circulation in the legs. To perform calf raises, stand with your feet hip-width apart and slowly rise onto your toes, lifting your heels off the ground. Hold for a moment before lowering back down. Repeat this movement for 10-15 repetitions, focusing on engaging your calf muscles.

For added challenge, you can perform calf raises on the edge of a step, allowing for a deeper stretch in the calves. This exercise enhances blood circulation, supports lymphatic drainage, and strengthens the lower legs. Make calf raises a part of your daily routine to promote overall leg health.

Low Squat for Lymph Nodes in Legs

The Low Squat pose is effective for stimulating the lymph nodes in the legs. Begin by standing with your feet slightly wider than hip-width apart. Slowly lower your body into a squat position, keeping your heels on the ground if possible. Hold this position for 30 seconds, breathing deeply to encourage relaxation.

To enhance the benefits, you can gently press your elbows against your inner thighs to deepen the stretch. This pose not only targets the lymph nodes but also improves flexibility in the hips and legs. Practice Low Squat regularly to support lymphatic health and improve overall lower body strength

Feet Circles to Release Ankle Tension

Feet circles are a great way to release tension in the ankles and promote circulation. Sit comfortably with your legs extended in front of you. Lift one foot off the ground and make small circles with your toes, rotating in one direction for 10-15 repetitions before switching directions. Repeat this process with the other foot.

To enhance the exercise, you can perform feet circles while standing or use a resistance band around your feet for added resistance. This simple movement encourages fluidity in the joints, promotes lymphatic flow, and helps relieve tension in the ankles. Incorporate feet circles into your routine for better ankle mobility and overall leg health.

CHAPTER 8:

Detoxifying with Twists and Inversions

Benefits of Twisting for Detoxification

Twisting poses in yoga are believed to enhance detoxification by stimulating the internal organs, particularly the liver and kidneys. When you twist, you create compression and release on these organs, which helps to expel toxins and promote better digestion. This process can also improve blood circulation, ensuring that the body efficiently eliminates waste.

Moreover, twisting poses encourage the movement of lymph fluid, which is crucial for maintaining a healthy immune system. By incorporating regular twisting sequences into your yoga practice, you can support your body's natural detoxification processes, leaving you feeling rejuvenated and energized.

Seated Twist to Promote Spinal Mobility

To perform a seated twist, start in a comfortable seated position with your legs crossed. Inhale deeply, lengthening your spine, and as you exhale, place your right hand behind you on the floor and your left hand on your right knee. Gently twist your torso to the right while keeping your spine straight. Hold this position for several breaths, then switch sides.

This pose not only enhances spinal mobility but also engages your core muscles. By focusing on your breath during the twist, you can deepen the stretch and improve your overall flexibility, making it an excellent practice for beginners.

Reclined Twist for Overall Relaxation

Begin by lying on your back with your knees bent and feet flat on the floor. Slowly drop your knees to one side while extending your arms out to a T-shape. Turn your head to the opposite side, allowing your body to relax into the twist. Hold this position for five to ten breaths before switching sides.

This pose is perfect for releasing tension in the lower back and promoting relaxation throughout the entire body. It's an excellent way to unwind after a long day, as it encourages deep breathing and mindfulness.

Supine Spinal Twist for Deeper Stretch

Start by lying on your back with your knees drawn to your chest. Slowly lower both knees to one side while keeping your shoulders pressed into the ground. Extend your arms out to the sides and gaze in the opposite direction of your knees. Hold this position for several breaths and then switch sides.

The supine spinal twist provides a deeper stretch for the spine and hips, which can alleviate tightness and discomfort. Focus on breathing deeply into your abdomen, allowing your body to release tension with each exhale.

Inversions for Head and Neck Lymph Flow

Inversion poses like Downward Dog or Shoulder Stand can significantly improve lymphatic drainage in the head and neck. To practice Downward Dog, start on all fours, then lift your hips up and back, forming an inverted "V" shape with your body. Hold the position for several breaths, letting your head hang freely.

Inversions allow gravity to assist in the movement of lymph fluid, promoting detoxification and relieving pressure in the upper body. Regular practice can help reduce headaches and improve overall well-being.

Shoulder Stand to Enhance Lymph Drainage

To perform the Shoulder Stand, lie on your back and lift your legs overhead, supporting your lower back with your hands. Keep your elbows close together, and ensure your weight is on your shoulders, not your neck. Hold this pose for several breaths, focusing on your breath as you engage your core.

This pose helps to stimulate the lymphatic system in the neck and shoulders, promoting detoxification. It's essential to practice this pose with caution and ensure proper alignment to avoid strain or injury.

Legs-Up-the-Wall Pose for Easy Inversion

Find a wall and sit with one side of your body against it. Swing your legs up the wall as you lie back on the floor. Your body should form an L-shape. Relax your arms by your sides and hold this position for 5-15 minutes, focusing on your breath.

This restorative pose encourages lymphatic drainage and reduces swelling in the legs. It's a gentle way to experience inversion benefits without strain, making it accessible for beginners and those with limited flexibility.

Gentle Back Twists for Safety

For a gentle back twist, sit cross-legged or in a chair. Inhale to lengthen your spine, and as you exhale, slowly twist to one side, placing your hand on your opposite knee for support. Hold this position for a few breaths before switching sides.

Gentle back twists are ideal for those new to yoga or with limited mobility. They allow for safe exploration of twisting while still promoting spinal health and flexibility without the risk of injury.

Forward Fold Twist for Variation

Start in a standing position and hinge at your hips to fold forward. Place one hand on the ground and rotate your torso, reaching the opposite arm toward the ceiling. Hold this position for several breaths before switching sides.

The forward fold twist combines a deep stretch for the hamstrings with the benefits of twisting. This pose enhances spinal mobility while allowing for variations that can be adapted to individual flexibility levels.

Yoga Block Usage for Support in Twists

Incorporating yoga blocks can provide additional support and stability during twisting poses. For example, in a seated twist, you can place a block under your hand for extra height, allowing you to maintain proper alignment and deepen the twist.

Using blocks helps beginners feel more secure in their poses, enabling them to focus on breath and movement without strain. This modification can make challenging poses more accessible and enjoyable.

How Twisting Releases Toxins

Twisting poses create a massage-like effect on internal organs, particularly the digestive organs, promoting the release of built-up toxins. As you twist, the compression and subsequent release help to improve blood flow and stimulate the lymphatic system, facilitating detoxification.

Additionally, by enhancing circulation, twisting poses allow fresh oxygen-rich blood to nourish your organs while expelling waste products. This dual action is vital for overall health and vitality, making twisting a key component of a detoxifying yoga practice.

Pairing Twists with Breathing Exercises

To maximize the benefits of twisting poses, pair them with deep breathing exercises. For instance, as you twist, inhale deeply to lengthen your spine and expand your ribcage, then exhale as you deepen the twist. This rhythmic breathing enhances oxygen flow and supports the detoxification process.

Incorporating breathing techniques like Ujjayi breath during twists can help to focus your mind and deepen your practice. This combination fosters a more profound sense of relaxation and clarity, making the experience more beneficial.

Safety in Twisting Poses

When practicing twisting poses, it's essential to prioritize safety to prevent injury. Always warm up with gentle stretches before attempting twists, and listen to your body. Avoid forcing the twist; instead, move into it gradually and maintain proper alignment.

CHAPTER 9:

Developing a Personalized Practice Routine

Understanding Personal Goals for Lymphatic Health

Before starting a yoga practice focused on lymphatic health, it's essential to identify your personal goals. Reflect on what you want to achieve, whether it's improving circulation, reducing swelling, or enhancing detoxification. Take some time to journal your current health status and any symptoms you experience related to lymphatic dysfunction. This self-assessment will help guide your practice and ensure it meets your specific needs.

Once your goals are established, consider how these align with your lifestyle. Are you looking for a gentle routine or a more vigorous practice? Setting clear, attainable goals will not only provide direction but also make your yoga journey more meaningful. Discuss your goals with a yoga instructor knowledgeable in therapeutic practices to tailor your sessions effectively.

How to Build a Custom Sequence

Creating a custom yoga sequence tailored to lymphatic health involves selecting poses that stimulate lymphatic flow. Begin with gentle stretches and restorative postures, such as legs-up-the-wall (Viparita Karani) and supported bridge pose (Setu Bandhasana). These poses promote drainage and enhance circulation in the lower body. You can also include twists, like seated spinal twists (Ardha Matsyendrasana), which help massage internal organs and stimulate lymphatic flow.

When building your sequence, aim for a balanced mix of restorative and invigorating poses. Start with a warm-up to prepare your body, then progress through your selected postures, and finish with a calming cool-down. Keeping a written sequence or using a yoga app can help you stay organized and focused on your goals, allowing you to adjust as necessary.

Setting a Daily Practice Time

Establishing a consistent daily practice time is crucial for developing a habit and improving lymphatic health. Choose a time that fits comfortably into your routine, whether it's early morning, midday, or evening. Setting a specific time each day helps signal to your body that it's time to practice, making it easier to prioritize your well-being.

To reinforce this habit, create a conducive environment for your practice. Designate a quiet space in your home, free from distractions, and gather your yoga props. Setting an alarm or reminder can also help you stick to your practice schedule, turning your daily yoga into a rewarding ritual rather than a chore.

Balancing Upper and Lower Body Poses

Incorporating a balance of upper and lower body poses is essential for a holistic approach to lymphatic health. Start your practice with lower body poses, such as forward bends (Uttanasana) or gentle lunges, to promote drainage and circulation in the legs. Afterward, transition to upper body poses like gentle shoulder openers (e.g., cow face arms) and heart openers (e.g., bridge pose) to encourage lymphatic flow in the upper body.

Aim to include poses that engage multiple muscle groups, promoting overall balance and coordination. By focusing on both upper and lower body poses, you create a well-rounded practice that enhances lymphatic drainage and supports the body's detoxification processes.

Combining Breathwork with Poses

Integrating breath work into your yoga practice can significantly enhance its effectiveness for lymphatic health. Begin with simple pranayama techniques, such as diaphragmatic breathing or alternate nostril breathing (Nadi Shodhana). These practices help to reduce stress and increase oxygen flow to your cells, which is vital for lymphatic function.

As you progress through your poses, synchronize your breath with movement. Inhale deeply as you expand into a pose, and exhale slowly as you relax into it. This mindful breathing will not only deepen your practice but also stimulate lymphatic circulation, making each movement more intentional and impactful.

Adding Mindfulness Practices

Incorporating mindfulness into your yoga practice is essential for fostering a deeper connection with your body and enhancing lymphatic health. Start by setting an intention before each session, focusing on how your body feels and what you wish to achieve. Consider practicing mindfulness meditation for a few minutes at the beginning or end of your session to cultivate awareness.

During your practice, pay close attention to sensations in your body. Notice areas of tension or discomfort, and consciously release these as you move through your poses. This heightened awareness can enhance your understanding of your body's needs, making your practice more effective in supporting lymphatic function.

Adjusting for Energy Levels

Listening to your body and adjusting your practice according to your energy levels is vital for maintaining a sustainable yoga routine. On days when you're feeling low energy, opt for restorative poses like child's pose (Balasana) or gentle seated stretches that promote relaxation and lymphatic flow without exertion.

Conversely, when you feel energized, incorporate more dynamic movements, such as sun salutations (Surya Namaskar) and standing poses, to stimulate your lymphatic system actively. This adaptability ensures your practice remains beneficial and enjoyable, preventing burnout while supporting your lymphatic health.

Techniques for Practicing at Home

Practicing yoga at home offers flexibility and convenience, allowing you to create a space that suits your needs. Start by designating a comfortable area where you can spread out your yoga mat and practice without interruptions. Use online resources, such as yoga videos or apps, to guide your sessions, especially if you're new to certain poses or sequences.

To maintain motivation, create a structured schedule for your home practice. Setting specific days and times for yoga, combined with journaling your experiences, can enhance your commitment and progress. Remember to keep your practice space inviting, perhaps with calming music or aromatherapy, to create an atmosphere conducive to relaxation and focus.

How to Use Yoga Props Effectively

Yoga props can enhance your practice by providing support and stability, especially for beginners or those with specific health concerns. Start with essentials like blocks, straps, and bolsters to help modify poses and maintain alignment. For example, using a block under your hands in forward folds can make the pose more accessible and comfortable.

Incorporate props into your routine gradually, exploring how they can assist in various poses. For instance, use a bolster in supported bridge pose to ease tension in the back or a strap for deeper stretches in hamstring poses.

Learning to use props effectively can enhance your practice and make it safer and more enjoyable.

Gradually Increasing Practice Duration

When establishing your yoga routine for lymphatic health, it's essential to gradually increase your practice duration to avoid overwhelm. Start with shorter sessions, perhaps 10 to 15 minutes, focusing on key poses and breath work. As you become more comfortable, aim to extend your practice by 5 to 10 minutes each week, incorporating new poses or sequences.

This gradual approach not only helps your body adapt but also builds confidence in your practice. Tracking your progress in a journal can provide motivation and insights into how your body responds to longer sessions, allowing you to tailor your routine further based on your comfort and energy levels.

Tips for Staying Motivated

Maintaining motivation in your yoga practice can be challenging, especially as time goes on. Set realistic and achievable goals that you can celebrate upon completion. This can include mastering a new pose or maintaining a consistent practice schedule for a month. Celebrating these milestones will keep your spirits high and encourage ongoing commitment.

Consider finding a yoga buddy or joining online communities focused on lymphatic health through yoga. Sharing your journey with others can provide support and accountability, making your practice feel less solitary. Additionally, exploring various styles of yoga or attending workshops can refresh your routine and reignite your passion for practice.

Weekly Check-Ins to Monitor Progress

Incorporating weekly check-ins into your yoga routine can help you assess your progress and make necessary adjustments. Set aside time each week to reflect on how you feel physically and emotionally after your practices. Journaling your experiences can help track changes in your lymphatic health, energy levels, and overall well-being.

During these check-ins, review your goals and see if they still align with your current needs. Adjust your practice or set new goals as necessary. This reflective process will not only keep you engaged but also deepen your understanding of your body's responses to your yoga practice.

Setting Achievable Milestones

Establishing achievable milestones within your yoga practice can provide motivation and a sense of accomplishment. Start with small, attainable goals, such as practicing three times a week or mastering a specific pose. These milestones serve as stepping stones to your larger objectives, making the journey feel manageable and rewarding.

As you achieve these smaller milestones, take time to acknowledge your progress. Celebrate your successes, no matter how minor, as they contribute to your overall journey toward better lymphatic health. This positive reinforcement will encourage continued dedication and enthusiasm for your practice.

Understanding Personal Goals for Lymphatic Health

Before starting a yoga practice focused on lymphatic health, it's essential to identify your personal goals. Reflect on what you want to achieve, whether it's improving circulation, reducing swelling, or enhancing detoxification. Take some time to journal your current health status and any symptoms you experience related to lymphatic dysfunction. This self-assessment will help guide your practice and ensure it meets your specific needs.

Once your goals are established, consider how these align with your lifestyle. Are you looking for a gentle routine or a more vigorous practice? Setting clear, attainable goals will not only provide direction but also make your yoga journey more meaningful. Discuss your goals with a yoga instructor knowledgeable in therapeutic practices to tailor your sessions effectively.

How to Build a Custom Sequence

Creating a custom yoga sequence tailored to lymphatic health involves selecting poses that stimulate lymphatic flow. Begin with gentle stretches and restorative postures, such as legs-up-the-wall (Viparita Karani) and supported bridge pose (Setu Bandhasana). These poses promote drainage and enhance circulation in the lower body. You can also include twists, like seated spinal twists (Ardha Matsyendrasana), which help massage internal organs and stimulate lymphatic flow.

When building your sequence, aim for a balanced mix of restorative and invigorating poses. Start with a warm-up to prepare your body, then progress through your selected postures, and finish with a calming cool-down. Keeping a written sequence or using a yoga app can help you stay organized and focused on your goals, allowing you to adjust as necessary.

Setting a Daily Practice Time

Establishing a consistent daily practice time is crucial for developing a habit and improving lymphatic health. Choose a time that fits comfortably into your routine, whether it's early morning, midday, or evening. Setting a specific time each day helps signal to your body that it's time to practice, making it easier to prioritize your well-being.

To reinforce this habit, create a conducive environment for your practice. Designate a quiet space in your home, free from distractions, and gather your yoga props. Setting an alarm or reminder can also help you stick to your practice schedule, turning your daily yoga into a rewarding ritual rather than a chore.

Balancing Upper and Lower Body Poses

Incorporating a balance of upper and lower body poses is essential for a holistic approach to lymphatic health. Start your practice with lower body poses, such as forward bends (Uttanasana) or gentle lunges, to promote drainage and circulation in the legs. Afterward, transition to upper body poses like gentle shoulder openers (e.g., cow face arms) and heart openers (e.g., bridge pose) to encourage lymphatic flow in the upper body.

Aim to include poses that engage multiple muscle groups, promoting overall balance and coordination. By focusing on both upper and lower body poses, you create a well-rounded practice that enhances lymphatic drainage and supports the body's detoxification processes.

Combining Breathwork with Poses

Integrating breath work into your yoga practice can significantly enhance its effectiveness for lymphatic health. Begin with simple pranayama techniques, such as diaphragmatic breathing or alternate nostril breathing (Nadi Shodhana). These practices help to reduce stress and increase oxygen flow to your cells, which is vital for lymphatic function.

As you progress through your poses, synchronize your breath with movement. Inhale deeply as you expand into a pose, and exhale slowly as you relax into it. This mindful breathing will not only deepen your practice but also stimulate lymphatic circulation, making each movement more intentional and impactful.

Adding Mindfulness Practices

Incorporating mindfulness into your yoga practice is essential for fostering a deeper connection with your body and enhancing lymphatic health. Start by setting an intention before each session, focusing on how your body feels and what you wish to achieve. Consider practicing mindfulness meditation for a few minutes at the beginning or end of your session to cultivate awareness.

During your practice, pay close attention to sensations in your body. Notice areas of tension or discomfort, and consciously release these as you move through your poses. This heightened awareness can enhance your understanding of your body's needs, making your practice more effective in supporting lymphatic function.

Adjusting for Energy Levels

Listening to your body and adjusting your practice according to your energy levels is vital for maintaining a sustainable yoga routine. On days when you're feeling low energy, opt for restorative poses like child's pose (Balasana) or gentle seated stretches that promote relaxation and lymphatic flow without exertion.

Conversely, when you feel energized, incorporate more dynamic movements, such as sun salutations (Surya Namaskar) and standing poses, to stimulate your lymphatic system actively. This adaptability ensures your practice remains beneficial and enjoyable, preventing burnout while supporting your lymphatic health.

Techniques for Practicing at Home

Practicing yoga at home offers flexibility and convenience, allowing you to create a space that suits your needs. Start by designating a comfortable area where you can spread out your yoga mat and practice without interruptions. Use online resources, such as yoga videos or apps, to guide your sessions, especially if you're new to certain poses or sequences.

To maintain motivation, create a structured schedule for your home practice. Setting specific days and times for yoga, combined with journaling your experiences, can enhance your commitment and progress. Remember to keep your practice space inviting, perhaps with calming music or aromatherapy, to create an atmosphere conducive to relaxation and focus.

How to Use Yoga Props Effectively

Yoga props can enhance your practice by providing support and stability, especially for beginners or those with specific health concerns. Start with essentials like blocks, straps, and bolsters to help modify poses and maintain alignment. For example, using a block under your hands in forward folds can make the pose more accessible and comfortable.

Incorporate props into your routine gradually, exploring how they can assist in various poses. For instance, use a bolster in supported bridge pose to ease tension in the back or a strap for deeper stretches in hamstring poses. Learning to use props effectively can enhance your practice and make it safer and more enjoyable.

Gradually Increasing Practice Duration

When establishing your yoga routine for lymphatic health, it's essential to gradually increase your practice duration to avoid overwhelm. Start with shorter sessions, perhaps 10 to 15 minutes, focusing on key poses and breathwork. As you become more comfortable, aim to extend your practice by 5 to 10 minutes each week, incorporating new poses or sequences.

This gradual approach not only helps your body adapt but also builds confidence in your practice. Tracking your progress in a journal can provide motivation and insights into how your body responds to longer sessions, allowing you to tailor your routine further based on your comfort and energy levels.

Tips for Staying Motivated

Maintaining motivation in your yoga practice can be challenging, especially as time goes on. Set realistic and achievable goals that you can celebrate upon completion. This can include mastering a new pose or maintaining a consistent practice schedule for a month. Celebrating these milestones will keep your spirits high and encourage ongoing commitment.

Consider finding a yoga buddy or joining online communities focused on lymphatic health through yoga. Sharing your journey with others can provide support and accountability, making your practice feel less solitary. Additionally, exploring various styles of yoga or attending workshops can refresh your routine and reignite your passion for practice.

Weekly Check-Ins to Monitor Progress

Incorporating weekly check-ins into your yoga routine can help you assess your progress and make necessary adjustments. Set aside time each week to reflect on how you feel physically and emotionally after your practices. Journaling your experiences can help track changes in your lymphatic health, energy levels, and overall well-being.

During these check-ins, review your goals and see if they still align with your current needs. Adjust your practice or set new goals as necessary. This reflective process will not only keep you engaged but also deepen your understanding of your body's responses to your yoga practice.

Setting Achievable Milestones

Establishing achievable milestones within your yoga practice can provide motivation and a sense of accomplishment. Start with small, attainable goals, such as practicing three times a week or mastering a specific pose. These milestones serve as stepping stones to your larger objectives, making the journey feel manageable and rewarding.

As you achieve these smaller milestones, take time to acknowledge your progress. Celebrate your successes, no matter how minor, as they contribute to your overall journey toward better lymphatic health. This positive reinforcement will encourage continued dedication and enthusiasm for your practice.

Common Concerns and Detailed FAQs

Can Lymphatic Yoga Benefit My Immune Health?

Lymphatic yoga can significantly enhance immune health by promoting lymphatic circulation, which is essential for detoxifying the body. The lymphatic system helps remove waste, toxins, and excess fluids, allowing your immune system to function more effectively. Incorporating gentle movements and breath work stimulates lymph flow, encouraging the body to eliminate waste and reduce inflammation.

To experience these benefits, include poses such as downward dog, shoulder bridge, and seated twists in your routine. Focus on deep, rhythmic breathing during each pose to further activate lymphatic drainage. Consistent practice can lead to improved immune response, helping you feel more energized and resilient against illness.

How Often Should I Practice for Best Results?

For optimal results, aim to practice lymphatic yoga at least three to four times a week. Regular practice encourages consistent lymphatic flow and supports the body's natural detoxification processes. Each session can last from 30 minutes to an hour, allowing ample time to move through various poses and integrate deep breathing techniques.

Start with shorter sessions if you're new to yoga, gradually increasing the duration as you become more comfortable. Listen to your body; finding a frequency that suits your lifestyle and energy levels is essential for **establishing a sustainable practice.**

Are There Any Contraindications for Lymphatic Yoga?

While lymphatic yoga is generally safe, some individuals should exercise caution. Contraindications include active infections, severe swelling, or acute conditions such as blood clots. If you have any underlying health conditions or concerns, consult with a healthcare professional before starting a lymphatic yoga practice.

Always be aware of your body's signals. If you experience any unusual symptoms during practice, such as severe pain or excessive fatigue, stop and reassess. Adjust your routine as needed to ensure a safe and beneficial experience.

What If I Experience Discomfort in Poses?

Experiencing discomfort during yoga is common, especially if you're new to the practice. To manage discomfort, focus on proper alignment and ensure you're not pushing yourself into poses. Utilize props, like blocks or bolsters, to support your body and modify poses as needed.

If discomfort persists, it may be beneficial to consult with a certified yoga instructor. They can offer personalized guidance and adjustments to help you safely navigate the poses, ensuring a more comfortable practice while still reaping the benefits of lymphatic yoga.

Is Lymphatic Yoga Suitable for All Ages?

Lymphatic yoga can be adapted for all ages, making it accessible to everyone, from children to seniors. The gentle movements and breath-focused techniques can support overall wellness and vitality, regardless of age or fitness level. Tailoring poses to individual capabilities is crucial, allowing for safe and effective practice.

For older adults or those with mobility issues, consider starting with chair yoga or gentle floor routines. Engaging in community classes or online tutorials can also provide guidance, ensuring that you find suitable modifications and foster confidence in your practice.

Conclusion

By embracing yoga techniques that focus on lymphatic health, beginners can safely promote their body's natural detoxification and immunity enhancement. This journey encourages not only physical improvement but also mental clarity, providing a comprehensive approach to wellness through dedicated practice.

www.ingramcontent.com/pod-product-compliance
Lightning Source LLC
Chambersburg PA
CBHW071029250726
48653CB00005B/1780